Opportunities in the
TRILLION DOLLAR
Wellness Industry

Opportunities in the

TRILLION DOLLAR

Wellness Industry

SELVA SUGUNENDRAN

CEng, MIEE, MCMI, CHt, MIMDHA, MBBNLP, MABNLP

#1 Best Selling Author, Speaker &
"Success Through Wellness" Coach

To order additional copies of this book, contact:
Xlibris Corporation
0-800-644-6988
www.xlibrispublishing.co.uk
Orders@xlibrispublishing.co.uk
303644

Contents

Dedication

This book is dedicated to my late mother Violet Ratnam for instilling in me the importance of prevention over treatment and my late father Morrison Selva Ratnam for teaching the disciplines necessary to take on and be successful in any challenge I undertook.

Acknowledgements

First of all, I would like to acknowledge the following people who have indeed paved the way for this explosive growth in the Wellness Industry. They have inspired me and their work has enabled me to write this book so that more people will be able to lead healthier, happier and longer lives, while becoming wealthier and successful in the process.

These great men include J.I. Rodale, Dr. James L Chestnut, Steve Demos, Carl F. Rehnborg, Frank Yanowitzand lastly but most importantly Paul Zane Pilzer whose contribution has enriched my life and energized me to write this book with full conviction.

Finally and most importantly, I wish to give thanks to my family. I thank my wife for her support and understanding as I spent long hours researching and travelling to gather the required data to write this book. My thanks go to my mother for instilling in me the importance of prevention over treatment and my father for teaching the disciplines necessary to take on and be successful in any challenge I undertook.

My thanks also go to my son Shaun and daughter (in-law) Florence for giving and sharing the love and joy of my two grand children, Jason and Lisa. Jason at just 4 years old also provides the inspiration I need with his own creativity, positive outlook and analytical mind.

SELVA SUGUNENDRAN
CEng, MIEE, MCMI, CHt, MIMDHA, MBBNLP, MABNLP

I also wish to say a huge thank you to my lovely niece Samantha Manoharan for always managing to find the time to check (for errors) the hundreds of articles that I have published during the last two years.

I cannot end this acknowledgement without giving thanks to God who has provided me with everything I need as illustrated in Philippians 4:verses 11-13.

Prologue

By opening this book you have started the journey of becoming a part of a trillion dollar industry in the making—the wellness industry.

Some of you who are reading this book might have read the other two books in my series of books on *How To Become Healthier, Wealthier and Successful Through Moving From Sickness to Wellness Solutions,* so you might have an idea of what the wellness industry is and how it is changing the world . . . one day at a time. However, for those of you who haven't I'd like to take this time to educate you about the basics of the wellness industry.

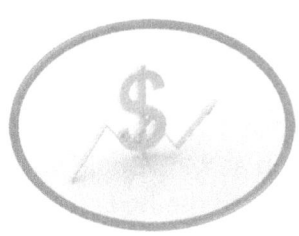 The wellness industry is a trillion dollar industry in the making. Years and years ago people didn't give a second thought about their wellness, their health or their well being. Not necessarily because they didn't care, but because we as people were not as educated.

Think about it—in the 1930's it was the 'in' thing to smoke cigarettes. Everyone including mothers and even children at the tender age of 12 smoked. Back then we didn't realize just how harmful cigarette smoke was, how it could cause lung cancer or any other cancer for that matter; we didn't know what we were putting in our bodies, and we didn't know how bad those toxins were.

However, as we grew and learned, we started to find that cigarettes are extremely harmful and hazardous to our health.

This is exactly the reason why the wellness industry is continuing to grow. As we become more educated about food, our bodies, toxins and how we can prolong our youth and our life, we naturally become more devoted to our health—hence the reason why the wellness industry is becoming the *trillion dollar wellness industry*.

Over the last two decades things really started to change as we as people began to actually *care* about our wellness, our quality of life and our youth. People are learning that exercise, eating right and dedication to their well being is extremely important. This means that we choose to eat right, take vitamins, exercise and that we search to find other natural ways to take care of ourselves. Wellness doesn't mean "New Age" nonsense.

For example, back in the day the only way that one could really have a good, healthy solid meal was to make it themselves. Restaurants were not necessarily known to provide healthy alternatives to their favorite dishes.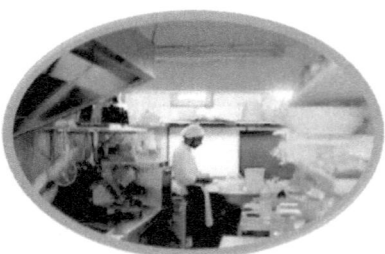

Today, the wellness revolution is being embraced by restaurants across the globe—even fast food restaurants such as McDonalds are jumping on board. They offer healthier alternatives to their traditional *Big Mac*, by selling salads and other options.

Whole Foods shops, natural or organic produce and meat, as well as vitamins and minerals are also becoming quite popular in today's society. People are striving to do better for themselves, striving to be as healthy as possible, striving to educate themselves about their own wellness and the wellness of others and how they can continue on the path. This is another reason why the wellness industry will continue to grow.

If you are someone who is devoted to wellness or at least someone who would *like* to be in the near future it is best to educate yourself. Once you become a bit knowledgeable you can also jump on board and join the revolution! You will find that you can become rich in knowledge and wealth when it comes to this industry and you will change people's lives. Not only that, you can save people thousands and thousands of dollars by educating them about the wellness industry.

How?

Well, the wellness industry is something that in many ways should replace much of the medical illness and health industry. Not necessarily health insurance, but the percentage of money that is put in it. Individuals who are healthy and pay out large amounts of money each year to their health insurance so that they can have coverage [even if they don't go to the doctor—ever] are basically throwing away their money. Their employer is taking hundreds of dollars away from them each month *just in case they happen to get sick*. This is outrageous, because if employees are devoted to their wellness they will also find that they do not need to pay out that kind of money—that the wellness industry can save them money.

This is another reason why there are so many different opportunities for success within the wellness industry. The opportunities are practically endless, actually.

Throughout my series of books about *How To Become Healthier, Wealthier and Successful Through Moving From Sickness to Wellness Solutions* you will learn about what you can do to become successful in this industry, what is wrong with the sickness industry and how you can save money without devoting your time and money to it and so on.

If you would like more information you can also go to my website at *www.successthroughwellnessbooks.com*. Here you will find a ton of information that can be used to change your life, and the life of others.

Thank you in advance for reading this book and my series of other wellness related books and articles. My hope is that I am able to reach my audience in some ways, bettering their life—even if in a small way. The *trillion dollar wellness industry* has changed my life for the better, which means it can change your life as well.

Wishing you the best, always!

Selva Sugunendran

Enter the Wellness Revolution

The Low Down on Pharmaceutical Companies and Why There Are So Many Opportunities for Success in Wellness

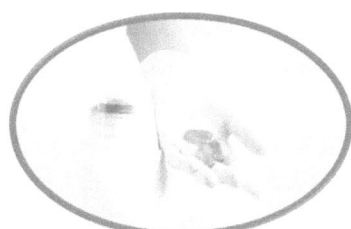 As appalling as it might sound, for the past three decades the majority of private R&D dollars in the pharmaceutical industry have been spent on products that treat the *symptoms of a disease rather than cure or prevent it.*

This, obviously, is something that creates permanent customers—and boosts the economy when someone needs to pay for a particular prescription that costs $200 because insurance won't cover it—month after month, for the rest of their lives.

The truth is, so many of the drugs out there do not even have a strong legitimate reason to be considered a prescription. They aren't addictive or controlled substances, so why can't they be sold over the counter? Well, they are issued in prescription form partly to get all Americans to subsidize 50 percent of their cost through tax deductions and to partly force employers to pay for them.

Not only that—and more importantly—many prescription drugs were designed to make you that wonderful customer for life although many prescription drugs are indirectly dangerous if you use them for life. Drugs like Lipitor, Zorcor, Nexium, Prevacid and Zoloft are the top-selling prescription drugs in the world.

They account for more than $25 billion in sales in the United States. That is a huge number, isn't it? Of course it is! And why would the medical or pharmaceutical industry want to lose that? They wouldn't—hence the reason for high priced prescription plans and insurance coverage.

These medications are also usually used long term—throwing away money that could be saved if the patient became more educated about the wellness industry and how they can start saving money. These particular drugs only *treat the symptoms of a particular illness*, ensuring that the medicine should be taken for the rest of someone's life. However, the drugs are not narcotics or controlled substances, so why are they on prescription? Again, to make more money.

The really bad thing about these drugs is that they are actually dangerous to your long-term health. How, you might ask? Well, think about it. As you continually take these drugs you are treating the symptoms of a disease. Therefore, these medications prevent you from actually modifying your behavior to cure the disease. So in many ways you could even be better off without the drugs *or finding an alternative.*

If you are someone who needs to take medications like these, there are a wide variety of alternatives out there—alternatives that just might actually treat the problem, instead of just masking the symptoms and giving you comfort.

If you are someone who is interested in investing in the wellness industry or starting your own business you will need to educate yourself in regards to the different remedies, products and services that just might make a difference in your life, as well as the life of your customers.

There is a great example that can be used, especially when it comes to the natural way to move away from using acid reducers such as Prevacid or Protonix. Millions of people in the United States suffer from some kind of indigestion—some more extreme [GERD] than others—that is treated with medicines such as these. Well, treated isn't necessarily the correct word because people who are prescribed these medications are usually stuck taking them for the rest of their lives, because if they stop taking the medication the symptoms persist.

Other examples include Essiac Tea or 'Floressence', which is a herbal tea that has been known to heal digestive issues and [in some case] minimize the size of cancerous tumors and/or cysts. The success of this wellness tea has been highly respected and known within the industry, but it is one that will not be acknowledged by the medical world.

Why?

The medical community would see a rapid decline in their economy which is why no one has been prepared to speak out saying that many natural remedies actually work.

There are tons of opportunities for entrepreneurs to grow their business within the wellness industry whether they are offering various products and services, classes and so on. The entrepreneurs who created and manufactured the products above have helped others and they have also become extremely successful within their business. This, however, is something that anyone can do through manufacturing or even distributing wellness products and services.

*   *   *

Throughout the rest of this book I will be discussing how you can take advantage of the wellness industry and join the revolution. With anyone—including your potential customers—you will always need to remain educated. If you aren't it will be very difficult for you to speak about your experience or even help others change their lives. In many ways it takes firsthand experience to really set forth on the path of wellness, especially for those you would like as long term customers or even for yourself. Why? Because many people have yet to have their first positive wellness experience. Once they do have this experience, though, they will [most likely] become a long-term wellness-focused individual.

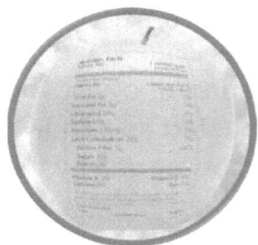 For instance, a woman in her mid-fifties was asked to change her diet by a wellness professional or doctor. So, she has chosen to eat healthier, but she has also decided to eat all-natural, organic food. Once she starts to eat organic or all-natural food she finds that she is feeling better and even *healthier* on a regular basis.

For instance, perhaps she has more energy and is no longer tired throughout the day. As you probably know firsthand, staying alert and motivated throughout the day is quite hard, especially when 2 o' clock in the afternoon hits. Some of us might resort to drinking Red Bull energy drinks, espresso or coffee, which can actually be a shock to our system if done frequently. However, when we start eating right, exercising and taking care of ourselves on a regular basis we will notice a world of difference with our energy levels and how we feel in general!

The way we feel on a regular basis does have a lot to do with diet, regardless of what one might think. This particular woman realizes that and quickly becomes entirely wellness-focused. She is now taking vitamins and minerals, as well as eating natural food. She has started that journey so now she will probably be a long term customer.

Homeopathic doctors are becoming increasingly popular as well. These are doctors who focus solely on homeopathic remedies for the mind, body and spirit. This could include meditations, natural detoxification of the body through colon cleanses and so on. There are even machines that these homeopathic doctors use in order to rid the body of hazardous toxins.

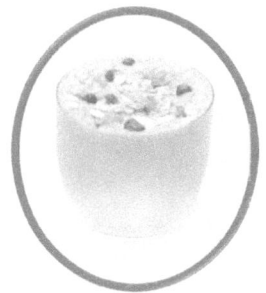

They can also recommend different herbal remedies for your specified symptoms—remedies that will [in many cases] be much cheaper than medically prescribed medication.

For anyone who has shopped at their nearest Whole Foods store, it is obvious that some natural remedies do cost a pretty penny. However, investing in your wellness is worth it because much of those remedies will help to actually cure the particular illness that you are experiencing, instead of merely covering it up or temporarily taking away the awful feelings you might be experiencing.

The example mentioned often goes hand in hand with any individual that experiences a positive result from something within the wellness industry. Once we feel better as a person, have more energy and actually *feel healthy* it is more than likely that we will not need to visit the doctor as often, which can save us [and our family] more money in the long run. Soon enough the entire family will join the wellness revolution, which will bring in even more customers for that particular business or entrepreneur.

Why?

Everyone on the face of the planet wants to feel good. They want to feel energized, healthy, alert and ready for every passing day. Not only that, as we age many of us want to look as young as they feel, which is also where the world of wellness comes in. After all, if we truly take care of our body—from the inside out, we will look much younger and even feel younger, and full of energy.

It Worked For Them, It Can Work For You

Success in Wellness

Almost everyone has heard of stem cell research. Stem cell research is truly an amazing scientific advance that honestly holds great promise for wellness and anti-aging. For one person, in particular, it was also something that has brought success into his life—all while helping others come into wellness.

People have thought badly of stem cell research in the past thanks to bad publicity that stated certain stem cells are harvested from human embryos. This is disturbing to many, yes, but there are so many different types of stem cells and you know what? Most of those stem cells have *nothing to do with human embryos!*

If you are unfamiliar with what a stem cell is, a stem cell is quite different from any other cells found in living organisms because they 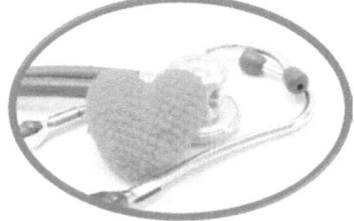 can divide *without limit*, replacing themselves and replenishing other cells. Stem cells are also based on their source such as adult, embryonic and bone marrow, and have three common characteristics.

Stem cells are capable of self-renewal, they are unspecialized and they can give rise to specialized cells, and the research can help individuals in so many different ways. One stem cell research in particular can help the health and wellness of our heart, which could potentially reduce heart disease. To many heart surgeons, heart surgery has been about mechanics. So, when something has failed in the heart, surgeons often go in and replace it physically with a mechanical device or a transplanted organ. Pig valves and pacemakers are so very common these days. In the past, few surgeons were well versed in stem cell biology and understood the implications behind the power of stem cells to heal and protect organs from damage.

Well, today [thanks to a stem cell researcher and a doctor named Dr. Reiss] researchers at Duke University have discovered that stem cells injected into the heart could *repair heart damage after a heart attack*. Stem cell research is a great progression in the world of medicine and one that [if continually researched] can make an even bigger difference in our lives and within the wellness industry. In the future it might be something that can stop the need for open heart surgery!

According to Dr. Reiss, medications and procedures can be critically important in the management of chronic disease, but they need to be recognized as adjuncts to one's personal wellness program. These wellness products can even save us money with our traditional healthcare because we will be healthier on a regular basis, minimizing the need to go to our medical provider, unless we need an annual exam or similar.

Even with stem cell research and other new procedures/research it is important for individuals to keep up with a healthy way of being to ensure that any procedure or remedy provides them with the best results possible. For instance, it wouldn't make much sense for a smoker to continue to run every single day of his life, five miles every morning, would it? No, because in actuality smoking while running can damage your lungs much faster than smoking without running. However, if you quit smoking and continue to run your lungs will improve and rejuvenate much, much faster.

With any kind of exercise, treatment or remedy it is always important to educate yourself [or those who are interested in that particular treatment] about any and all of the ways that they can better themselves and their lives. This is true in many different aspects in life because the more you become educated about a particular topic, the more versed you will become. So, even if it is a bit hard to dive into the wellness industry as a customer or even as an entrepreneur in the first instance, it will become a habit to either educate others about the industry and how they can better their lives and their whole body, mind and spirit, and how the wellness industry can thoroughly help you become rich.

The term "rich" does not necessarily mean *rolling in the dough*, it could also mean that you are rich with education in regards to your health, the health of others and how we [as people] can make a difference in the world we live in today by taking care of ourselves and others.

Obviously, if you are not a doctor it is not likely that you will come up with something like stem cell research. This doesn't mean that you will not be as successful in the *trillion dollar wellness industry* because there are thousands upon thousands of opportunities. Once you start learning about some of these opportunities it will become quite natural to discover more opportunities.

The wellness industry will continue to grow and flourish with opportunities, especially considering the fact that the individual cells in our body are constantly dying and replacing themselves. However, at one point in our life, regardless of who we are, something tells each cell in each bodily organ to stop reproducing itself—which is what causes normal aging or unwanted illnesses such as cancer.

The reason for the demand for wellness-based products and services, whether it is for vitamins, minerals, creams, oils, etc., is primarily driven by one function of code, the one that causes aging. Aging includes the wrinkles that appear on our face as well as the ultimate breakdown of our bodily organs. As we continue to evolve as people we proceed to understand and manipulate this code, ensuring that the wellness industry and its products continue to evolve as well.

Soon, based on the recently complete mapping of humans it should be possible to predict every forthcoming disease or condition not caused by external factors such as diet and exercise. Genetic testing to find out what type of diseases and illnesses we are susceptible to, thanks to our DNA, will soon be quite widespread as well. We will be able to figure out if someone is predisposed to cancer, osteoporosis and so on.

This being said, wellness professionals or entrepreneurs who actually embrace this emerging DNA-based technology first [in food and dietary areas] will see their business *explode with customers*. This is another reason why the wellness industry is the *trillion dollar industry*.

Eventually, vitamins and supplements used in this manner will be supplemented by genetic intervention especially when our technology proceeds to progress. With time we will most likely be able to modify or repair the gene that is giving us that illness or particular problem.

Much of the sickness related health industry will not accept this or push this to move forward, but soon enough the wellness industry will prove its worthiness to the traditional healthcare industry. Well, at least that is the hope. Scientists do not expect this type of intervention to become effective in treating the full spectrum of illness for a while, though—but it will happen.

Not only that, for individuals who are currently seeking natural ways to delay the progression of certain diseases, there are so many different products out there that have [in some cases] helped individuals overcome major illnesses—serious illness such as cancer or even controlling their diabetes. It's an interesting thought—actually overcoming or controlling an illness due to natural remedies from

SELVA SUGUNENDRAN
CEng, MIEE, MCMI, CHt, MIMDHA, MBBNLP, MABNLP

plants or roots that have been around for thousands of years, but it works and the world is beginning to see this.

Understanding these factors is what has made so many other individuals successful within the *trillion dollar wellness industry*. New wellness products are manufactured regularly. The thousands of products that are currently on the market will increase by the thousands within the next five years as well, which increases the potential for success!

In the first instance [before you decide whether or not you'd like to jump on the bandwagon] it is a good idea for you to educate yourself about a variety of different products and services that are out there. Once you have educated yourself you can then decide whether or not you'd like to become a distributor of products, a creator, manufacturer, small business owner and so on, because you will be able to decide just what you will be able to offer your potential customers.

For instance, I have a close friend of mine who started out on a wellness path herself because both of her children were on the autistic spectrum. She didn't want to give up hope for her two boys so she started to do some research on her own, finding that it has been proven that diet plays a huge role in autism as well as sickness or health based immunizations.

So, what did she do? She continued on with her education and started to only feed her children organic or all-natural food. Soon enough she was on the wellness revolution train taking homeopathic courses, reiki classes and a variety of other wellness-based endeavors. She decided that she wanted to ensure that her children were on all natural medications [not prescriptions], diets and so on. Now she is a very reputable homeopathic doctor that has continued on to help hundreds of customers each month.

She has opened up a small business that focuses on natural remedies for all illnesses, meditation, reiki, massage, detox programs and so on. Her vow to help her children transitioned into also helping herself and others. Again, once you really set out there and begin to make a difference you will feel rich in more ways than one.

Ways You Can Stake Your Claim to Wealth in the Wellness Industry

When it comes to the wellness industry there are a wide variety of ways that you can stake your claim to wealth as there are thousands upon thousands of opportunities. However, what about staking your claim as a non profit organization? To do good just for the sake of doing good? Interesting concept, right?

Sometimes a fortune can come by helping others, meaning that *you become rich by truly making a difference*. Sometimes this isn't monetarily! This doesn't mean, however, that monetary fortune cannot be enjoyed, though.

For instance, the wellness revolutionary Dr. Geoff Tabin set a personal goal to eliminate preventable blindness in his lifetime. You might be thinking that that is an awfully large goal, right? Well, it's a possibility because it is actually happening.

Consider the fact that 37 million people in the world are blind and 100 million people have low vision where they have a difficult time performing daily tasks or living, or working most jobs. The sad thing is that 85% of this blindness is *preventable or treatable*.

This is why Dr. Tabin decided to try to make a difference—any way that he could.

Around half of 137 million people suffer from curable cataracts, which is in all honesty the number one cause of blindness in the world today. A cataract is a clouding of the crystalline lens in the eye that affects *every human being if they live long enough.* So, how can this be curable? Well, there is a surgery called cataract surgery that removes the clouded lens, replacing it with an intraocular lens.

Cataract surgery is the most frequently performed surgery, with two million operations performed each year in the United States alone. This type of surgery is the most successful anti-aging or wellness treatment known to man, but the sad thing is—many people cannot have cataract surgery due to its cost. The cost is approximately $3,500 per eye and isn't covered by Medicare or most private health insurance.

Dr. Tabin knew that this surgery was extremely costly and that for those who could not afford the surgery, cataracts were a death sentence. Why? Because a blind family member could potentially be a great burden to family members. This is why Tabin dedicated himself to finding other affordable solutions that could help others such as opening the Tilganga Eye Center in 1994 as the first outpatient facility in the Himalayan region.

Today Dr. Tabin offers the surgery for $20USD. Obviously, the doctor has changed a lot of things when it comes to visual wellness, and the hope is that others will follow in his footsteps. It is possible to make a difference in someone's life—for the better.

If you are an investor [or someone who is looking to invest in a particular market] the wellness industry is actually a good choice. While the wellness industry is a *trillion dollar industry* it is important to become a customer of any company in which you are considering making an investment.

There is no substitute for using the products yourself when it comes to evaluating the long-term potential for a company, meaning that once you invest in a company and their products you want to ensure that you *inspect competitive products on a regular or periodic basis.*

Why?

Because the world of technology is also booming and it is always changing. It changes incredibly fast, so it is important to keep up with the times, because believe it or not it has a lot to do with businesses, their products and how well they do.

For instance, if you're a doctor or a wellness distributor, or even an insurance agent who is involved in the wellness industry somehow, you should always underwrite and evaluate the products of the companies within your specific industry. Yes, wellness is all about mind, body and spirit, but it is important that you keep up with your competitors. This is true for every single business out there.

This is called market and competitor research and it is important that you continuously keep up with your competitors and any other people that are in your industry. This will ensure that you understand or have some knowledge about what works for them, what doesn't and what you can do to improve your own business and the way you work to market or distribute your products.

For instance, you might find that starting weekly yoga classes in your business facility will increase how many regular customers you 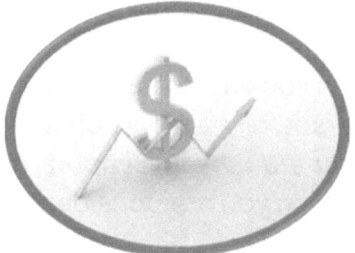 bring in, or even an educational program about vitamins, minerals or how your customers can better themselves by taking care of their mind, body and spirit might do the same. Eating right, dieting, exercising and the like is all included in this category.

As you can see, there is a wide variety of different things you can do to ensure that you as an investor are making a return on your investment. In all honesty, if the business you invest in does quite well on an annual basis it is likely that you will do quite well in turn. However, by completing marketing research and continuously striving for more you can become even more successful than you ever dreamed of.

Regardless of what you are interested in, you need to understand what area of the wellness industry you are interested in-manufacturing, distributing products and services, Direct Selling, or working as a practitioner.

For example, an accountant or banker could combine a wellness distribution with the opportunity to convert customers to wellness-oriented health insurance such as an HSA *or* just use that distribution to obtain more clients for their own accounting or banking business.

The same is equally true for a chef who learns how to make healthy versions of popular foods and then opens up his own *wellness restaurant*. They could also open a catering company or even become a wellness food manufacturer.

For instance, the chefs of the popular soy-based foods *Gardein* has also manufactured and distributed their products. They are so meat-like that they are becoming increasingly popular and they can be used in a variety of dishes, as seen at the popular restaurant The Yard House. The Yard House offers a wide of variety *Gardein* products such as chick'n pizza, bbq chick'n salad and so on. These meat alternatives have become increasingly popular, even among those individuals who are not entirely vegetarian, but who do not usually eat a lot of meat.

As another example, farmers or even home gardeners can start growing healthier foods like edamame and teach their customers how to use them. They can also create their own organic garden, keep their own chickens for organic eggs and even [if they want to go that far] raise deer or cattle and only keep their milk all-natural.

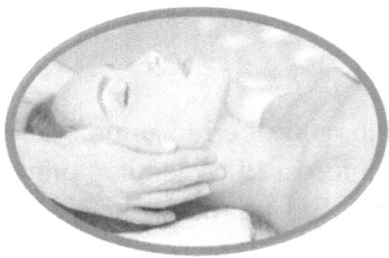

Massage therapists are in the ideal position to teach wellness and to begin distributing wellness products. As a massage therapist, you also have the chance to take your education a bit further and become a reiki practitioner, which is the next level of massage therapy. It is all about positive energy and healing your body naturally, and evening out your mind, body and spirit.

When it comes to herbal remedies, entrepreneurs and inventors and investors have discovered ways to even cure or treat illnesses that even the medical industry will not *treat*. Instead the medical industry will simply mask the symptoms or cover the symptoms so that they create a permanent customer for life—getting long-term payments from that individual. Soon enough, though, the wellness industry will be closely competing with the sickness industry and stepping on their tracks.

So, Why the Wellness Industry?

While I have not quite discussed every possible avenue available to take advantage of the *trillion dollar wellness industry*, I hope that you have come to realize just how beneficial the industry can be to you, your loved ones *and your quality of life*.

The wellness revolution is one that will change the lives of everyone that comes into contact with it—no matter who you are, what your background is or where you came from. This is equally true for those entrepreneurs or individuals who would like to set off and start creating their own wellness business. The opportunities are endless and life changing.

You can read through the rest of my books to learn more about the *trillion dollar wellness industry*, about what the medical or sickness industry has done absolutely wrong and how you can help change your life and the life of others. There are facts about the wellness and the sickness industry that go together, but my own personal hope is that people all across the globe will turn to wellness-oriented products and services in preference to sickness based solutions that treat symptoms only.

As an entrepreneur and wellness revolution leader I can tell you that the time is here to make a change. The time is here to enjoy your life as you were made to. There are no limits to what can be achieved and by following the wellness industry you will be able to [hopefully] prolong your existence as well, since you will be taking extra care of yourself.

You can imagine just how amazing it will be to be eating right, exercising and educating others about the wellness revolution on a regular basis. It's about living wellness, for sure.

Appendix

I have provided these articles as an appendix for you, as an added bonus. Enjoy!

What is Preventive Health Care?

As the old saying goes, prevention is better than cure. Thousands of individuals nowadays are looking for more ways to cut costs and avoid further complications by investing in wellness solutions or preventive health care. In medicine, earlier is always better, which is why people are encouraged to try a variety of remedies and routines that will ultimately keep them healthy and safe before any type of danger sets in. Knowing more about the approach will guide you properly on how to add years to your life.

Brief Description

Preventive health care or preventive medicine is described as taking the right measures that will keep diseases and injuries at bay, compared to having to cure and treat these and the associated symptoms. Preventive health care is a lot different compared to palliative and curative medicine. It focuses more on the specific needs of the individual, compared to generally providing regimens that counter various health problems. Primary prevention, however, is a population-based approach that can prevent epidemic and pandemic effects.

The Levels

There are 4 levels defined in wellness solutions, named primary, secondary, tertiary and quaternary. Primary prevention is described as taking measures that will prevent disease occurrence. Majority of health efforts focusing on entire populations are usually primary. Secondary prevention is described as approaches that identify or diagnose and treat current health problems during the early stages before it progresses to more serious complications. Tertiary prevention is defined as the methods that minimize the negative effects of present disease by reducing the complications and symptoms of the disease and restoring function. Quaternary prevention covers methods that will prevent results of excessive or unneeded practices in the health care system.

About Primal Prevention

Primal prevention is another term that defines all the necessary measures done to make sure that fetuses stay healthy and well-balanced to prevent further problems when they grow up. The measures are taken to prevent health conditions and diseases beginning from the gestation period. The approach is based on associations made between the well-being of the fetus or primal health and adult wellness and health. The methods for primal prevention usually involves providing information to parents about the drawback of epigenetic influences on the baby, parenting during infancy, financial help if needed and enough leave time for parents to take care of their children.

Things to Do

Preventive health care will include different techniques and methods, such as breastfeeding, handwashing and immunization. The health care system might also offer screening tests and programs that will cater to the patient, based on his current health status, medical and family history and age. For instance, individuals with a family history of diabetes or cancer should start checkups early on compared to people without such background. Preventive medicine also includes research and studies done by establishments and institutions that will enhance practices and help diagnose diseases and symptoms before these progress. There are various centers today that focus on specific health problems with the intent to treat the effects and symptoms before anything serious occurs.

Preventive Health Care: Scope and Practices

Preventive health care is proving to be more efficient and useful compared to sickness-based health care. More and more people and institutions are focusing on wellness solutions that try to delay or prevent illness compared to having to diagnose and treat a variety of problems that have already escalated due to poor health practices and prolonged lack of treatment. There are several ways to prevent disease from interrupting your lifestyle.

About Prophylaxis

Prophylaxis in Greek means "to guard" or "to prevent beforehand". It is defined as any public health or medical procedure with the intent to prevent diseases, instead of having to cure or treat. Prophylactic measures are generally divided between two types: primary prophylaxis and secondary prophylaxis. Primary prophylaxis means having to prevent the progression of a disease, while secondary prophylaxis means preventing the worsening of a disease that is already present in the person.

Prophylaxis Cases

There are many products and activities under the scope of prophylaxis. Vaccines are considered prophylactic, because these prevent people from suffering many diseases. Immunizations can even keep a person protected for life. Examples of vaccines are smallpox vaccine, polio vaccine, mumps vaccine, measles vaccine, HPV vaccine, influenza vaccine, hepatitis vaccine and many more. Many are provided during childhood or infancy, while new ones are also being developed, such as vaccines that prevent some cancers.

Other examples of prophylaxis include birth control approaches that can prevent sexually transmitted disease or STD and unwanted pregnancy. Examples of birth control methods are using condoms and taking contraceptive pills and medications. Physical exercise is also called prophylactic because it strengthens the entire body, especially the immune system. It's important to do some form of exercise regularly because it can prevent the occurrence of cancer, heart and cardiovascular problems, diabetes, skeletal problems, muscle ailments and several others.

More Prophylactic Cases

Teeth cleaning and fluoride therapy are also known as dental or oral prophylaxis, which should be done every 6 to 12 months. In some cases, antibiotics are considered as a form of prophylaxis, such as taking ciprofloxacin to prevent anthrax if an area is suspected to have an epidemic. TCAs or tricyclic antidepressants can prevent headache and migraine.

Polypill prevents cardiovascular illnesses. Heparin is used to prevent thrombosis among bedridden patients. Chloroquine and mefloquine are taken to prevent malaria. Potassium iodide is taken to prevent the development of thyroid cancer. Some surgeries are also considered preventive health care interventions, such as prophylactic mastectomies that lower the risk of breast cancer development among people with the mutation gene, BRCA.

Simpler Measures

Several actions are also known to prevent the occurence of disease and minimize the effects of an existing one, such as wearing masks and gloves when entering hospitals and other areas known to have contaminants. People should also wash their hands regularly since these harbor a lot of germs and disease-causing agents. Good hygiene will improve health significantly. People can also resort to other methods like eating a healthy diet, detoxification and stress-relief techniques that clear the system and mind.

Guidelines for Disease Prevention

Thousands of physicians and patients are quickly focusing more on wellness solutions or preventive health care for many good reasons. The approach is more sustainable and can provide more benefits compared to sickness-based methods that might only offer symptomatic treatment. Focusing on the health problem early on can lead to advantages that can last an entire lifetime. People can stay free of disease following these steps.

1. Stress-Relief and Rest

People should be aware that not getting enough rest can lead to health problems. Stress and lack of rest can weaken the immune system thereby making it more susceptible to disease and infection. It's important for children to get at least 10 to 12 hours of sleep everyday, while adults should aim for 7 or 8 at least. Stress-relief techniques are also very important because these rid the body of toxins and agents that can lead to illness. Some forms of stress-relief include yoga, meditation, deep breathing, visual imagery and taking short walks. Hitting the gym and cardiovascular exercise are also forms of stress-relief.

2. Maintain the Environment

Regularly clean your home and wipe off the surface of furniture and other items that are frequently used. Use a disinfectant when cleaning appliances, furniture, utensils, doors, telephones, faucet handles, and other surfaces in the house. Also get rid of the trash regularly. Check for presence of mold, bacteria and fungi in the house. Look for possible things that can trigger allergies, bacterial and viral growth and pain. If you have children in the house, make sure you baby-proof the environment to avoid accidents and injury.

3. Hygiene and Cross-Contamination

Good hygiene is one of the best ways to stay healthy and practice preventive health care. Wash your hands frequently, especially after coming into contact with places, things and people. Also take a bath at least once each day and brush your teeth regularly. Change dirty clothes and keep your shoes clean and smelling good. If you've been to a contaminated area like a hospital, it's best to leave your shoes outside the door and spray it with a disinfectant first. Avoid sharing things inside the house, such as toothbrushes, soaps, hats and shoes. You increase the chances of cross-contamination, thereby spreading a present disease to other members of the house.

4. Self-protection

Take a multivitamin everyday to boost your immune system. Also drink a lot of water to refresh the body and eliminate toxins and harmful agents. Try to stay away from sick people and minimize exposure especially to those suffering from serious ailments. Wear masks and gloves whenever possible and wash your hands afterwards. Also make use of other protective devices and products that prevent disease and injury, such as hard hats, condoms, vaccines, eyeglasses, etc.

5. Research

Having an idea about a possible outbreak or a current epidemic in your area will prepare you well on how to keep the disease at bay. You will know which pharmaceutical products to take to improve your immune system and quickly treat minor symptoms of the problem.

Preventive Health Care Vs. Sickness-Based Solutions

More groups are preferring wellness solutions or preventive health care over sickness-based solutions for various purposes. Primarily, finding means to take care of the problem before it even occurs is a cheaper and more effective way to save lives and promote health. Some types of diseases are also rendered incurable, so people diagnosed with health problems might have to live with the symptoms until death. Knowing the proper methods and comparing the differences will greatly help identify the pros and cons of each.

Prevention is Better Than Cure

Health experts and physicians wish to promote wellness solutions because it offers a wide array of methods that will ultimately avoid illness, as well as take care of people so that they don't have to deal with the effects of serious health problems. Sickness-based solutions focus more on the diagnosis and treatment of diseases that are already present. In some cases, it might already be too late for the individual if the disease has progressed to higher levels or has triggered other underlying conditions to start. The programs designed for disease are much easier to follow and can keep people free from sickness well into late adulthood. Programs for treatment of diseases can take many years, and can still lead to death even with the most advanced medications and technologies provided.

On Affordability

The cost of wellness solutions is a lot lower compared to treating current ailments. For example, having a healthier lifestyle will only require the person to initially consume healthier food, embark on a physical regimen and get more sleep each night. These almost do not change the budget or spending habits of individuals and can even lessen their expense each month. Purchasing multivitamins and other health boosters and herbal treatments is cheaper compared to buying medications for problems like diabetes or hypertension.

Changes in Lifestyle

Individuals who focus on wellness solutions will also find that the changes they make in themselves will actually provide balance to their lives. They will experience and enjoy the benefits of quitting smoking, alcohol and drugs. They also practice safety measures to keep protected from injuries and other known dangers. People that focus on sickness-based solutions are forced to change their lifestyle because they have already developed incapacities that might complicate the current disease. Embarking on an exercise program or dieting will only lead to minimal results and does not promise them full health afterwards.

Financial Opportunities

More companies are also investing in wellness solutions and preventive health care as people become more conscious of the effects of harmful agents and elements. There are plenty of multilevel companies offering health supplements, vitamins and minerals, beauty products, cosmetics, herbal supplements and energy boosters that offer to rid the body of toxins, as well as enhance the immune system. Regular individuals who try these products get the advantage of all-natural ingredients, plus they can also start their own business retailing the offerings. This is a lot different compared to bedridden patients that have to quit or limit their job because of current illness.

Preventive Health Care: The Risks and Causes

People will realize that wellness solutions or preventive health care is a lot cheaper and more effective compared to sickness-based solutions. Some diseases, once diagnosed, might be rendered incurable or can remain in the person for several months at a time. There is also the risk of relapse which can be a huge burden on the patient, as well as his family. Preventive measures will help keep symptoms and harsh effects at bay, as well as slow down or stop the progress of an underlying health condition.

Identifying the Risks

Before you embark in any preventive health care program, know more about the causes and risks involved so you can plan carefully. For conditions and cases that can still be helped by wellness solutions, hypertension is known to be the problem that leads to the most deaths, averaging 7.8 million each year. Smoking follows with 5 million deaths each year, then high cholesterol at 3.9 million. Other problems that increase mortality include malnutrition, sexually transmitted disease, unhealthy diet, obesity and being overweight, lack of exercise, alcohol, indoor air pollution, poor sanitation and unsafe water.

Risks in the United States

In the United States, preventable deaths are led by tobacco smoking, with 435,000 dying each year (18%). Living a sedentary lifestyle and unhealthy diet is second, causing 365,000 deaths. Alcohol consumption is third with 85,000 deaths per year. Other items that could possibly be avoided include infectious diseases, traffic collisions, toxicants, drug abuse, sexually transmitted disease and firearm cases.

Lowering Mortality

There are also known top preventive measures that boost health and prevent illness and disease among children ages 0 to 5 years old all over the globe. The most effective is breastfeeding, because natural mother's milk can provide colostrums to the baby. Colostrum is rich with disease-preventing agents that strengthen the person's immune system after birth. Breastfeeding prevents 13% of child deaths. The second effective method is treating materials with insecticide, preventing 7% of deaths, followed by complimentary feeding which lessens 6% of deaths. Other known methods include zinc intake, having clean delivery, Hib vaccination, good hygiene, sanitary and safe water, taking antenatal steroids, and proper control of newborn temperature. Infants should also be given vitamin A, tetanus toxoid vaccine, measles vaccine, antimalarial treatment during pregnancy, nevirapine, replacement feeding and antibiotics if membranes rupture prematurely.

Consumer Response

With all the risks and causes identified, people should become more aware and start practicing good health methods. Preventive health care is supported by various government bodies and medical institutions to lower and prevent cases before complications arise. The most basic things that people can do is right at home, by getting healthier food choices, adding exercise to their routine and sleeping better. They should also get immunized and mothers should be reminded about the importance of breastfeeding until the baby is 12 to 24 months. Signs, consumer warnings and labels should be read carefully and followed. Agencies should also make an effort to provide clean water and pollution-free environments for living places.

Preventive Health Care: The Way of the Future
Through Wellness health

Today, people no longer wish to wait until the disease occurs before finding possible treatments. Health is becoming a priority among thousands all around the world, which is why preventive health care (Wellness Health) is quickly becoming popular. There are also new products and companies emerging because of the need to stay disease-free and healthy for life ensuring wellness health. People should learn about the benefits and try the various methods to get the best results.

Recent Developments

One of the biggest fears that working individuals face is already happening. After the recent global recession and crisis, people can no longer rely on sickness-based systems to take care of them even after they have earned their financial protection and insurance policies. A lot of businesses have gone bankrupt and retirees are no longer secured the way people were several decades ago. Retirees have to keep working past the age of 65 years old just to make ends meet. More people are also unable to afford medical and hospitalization costs for different procedures, surgeries and medications.

Even with the fast growth and development of modern technology, especially in the health care sector, only a handful of individuals are able to pay for complete care and recovery. Some are forced to deal with their current health problems and diseases by compromising on medications and other interventions. People are now becoming more aware that sickness can add to the difficulties of their financial situation.

The Rise of Preventive Health Care—Wellness Health

Because of the problems mentioned above, companies and consumers are prioritizing the importance of preventive health care or wellness solutions. These approaches aim to identify the risk factors and encourage people to practice healthier lifestyles and invest in products and agencies that actually promote health, instead of having to deal with the consequences later. Getting rid of the risk factors and understanding the causes will greatly minimize cases, so people do not have to rely on ineffective systems.

Preventive health care is a fast-growing sector, estimated to earn billions of dollars each year within the next decade. Today, you will find several network marketing groups focusing on health supplements, nutritional food and drinks, vitamins and minerals and herbal products that cleanse the body, rid it of toxins and harmful agents and boost the immune system. Many of these products are not clinically approved but are scientifically tested with very viable results.

For the Consumers

In the next few years, preventive health care is viewed to either equal or overtake the need for diagnosis and treatment of diseases. People are planning to live healthier lives and are researching more on how to fight disease. Even those with current diseases can prevent progression and further complications. People should be aware that family history is a big source of information on what things they should expect. This allows them to take supplements and products that will lessen their susceptibility for developing cancer, diabetes, high blood pressure, etc.

The growth of businesses and agencies focusing on wellness solutions is also indicative that people understand the financial benefits that come with the health boost. Thousands of people are joining networks and starting their own online shops retailing health products and sharing preventive measures that will decrease morbidity and mortality rates.

Techniques for Preventive Health Care

Aside from the programs and recommendations provided by the government and health care sector, people can also independently practice preventive health care. They can start with the basics, quitting unhealthy habits and embarking on a diet and physical fitness regimen. Aside from getting rid of the risks and effects of disease, people can also boost health as a whole and add more years to their life. Stress can be relieved as well as other associated symptoms of a current or impending illness.

Initial Techniques

Everyone will recognize the benefits of eating the right food, exercising regularly and getting enough sleep each night. For dieters, people should make sure that they eat a balanced meal each day, consisting of all three food groups. People should avoid eating fried, sugary and fatty foods whenever possible. Also refrain from eating too many processed and refined goods. Try to aim for natural ingredients and pure forms of food. More and more individuals are getting organic and all-natural foods that provide health benefits and none of the effects that chemicals and preservatives offer.

Exercise Tips

When embarking on a physical regimen, start by doing exercises that you can realistically do without skipping workouts. Some people make the mistake of starting prevention health care by instantly overtraining, working out every single day, only to find that they're already too exhausted to continue after a week. If you have been sedentary for several months or years, start by working out 2 times a week, with each session lasting 30 to 45 minutes only. Use a combination of weight training and cardiovascular exercise.

Things to Avoid

Getting on a wellness solution program might also mean having to stop unhealthy practices that ruin your lifestyle and enhance the chances of developing disease. Some of the things you should quit include smoking, alcohol and drug abuse. Alcohol can still be taken but only in small or moderate amounts. Experts say that taking one glass of red wine or beer a night can actually be helpful in preventing some illnesses.

You should also refrain from overeating and practice proper intake of foods that can lead to high cholesterol, high blood pressure and diabetes. Others might decide to avoid activities that can lead to disease or injury, such as working in plastic factories, operating hazardous equipment or having jobs that are rated as highly risky.

Screening and Testing

Always make it a habit to do regular checkups and screening tests to determine the possibility of disease progressing in your body. There are several tests such as mammography, pap smear, breast self-examination, testicular self-examination, cholesterol screening, colon cancer screening, PSA test, CT scan, blood pressure and aortic ultrasound. Individuals should also be vigilant enough to check for physical signs and symptoms. Early warning signs can fully treat diseases. Check for lasting fever, lumps on the body, unexplained weight gain or loss, nonstop pains and aches in the body and chronic cough. Update your immunizations and research on current vaccines that you might not yet have been given.

The Advantages of Preventive Health Care

Thousands of individuals all over the globe are quickly becoming aware of the effects of globalization and how the modern era tends to be more dangerous to health and well-being. According to statistics, a lot of people in the United States are dying of preventable diseases caused by smoking, reckless driving, substance abuse and alcohol. Preventive health care can take care of all these by providing sufficient information and getting rid of the problem before it even starts. Knowing the bonuses will entice you to start immediately.

1. Staying Disease-Free

The main advantage that preventive health care or wellness solution offers is the possibility of staying free from disease and harmful symptoms. Instead of treating health problems that are already present, people are given the chance to live healthier lives, thus keeping the potential risks at bay. Some people can stay disease-free for life or can easily treat minor problems and risks. This is a lot better than having to treat problems that do not have known permanent cures like diabetes, cancer and heart ailments.

2. Targeting Several Health Problems

Preventive health care can be done to focus on specific health cases that the individual is likely to suffer. It can also be applied to prevent related and a wide array of other diseases. Experts will initially check the health history of patients to determine which conditions are usual in their background and can possibly develop over time, such as cancer, diabetes and cardiovascular disease. Doctors and health experts can then recommend a regimen and other supportive products that will reduce the risk of occurrence significantly. Improving your lifestyle will also free you from other potential problems, including the common cold, flu, malaria, liver disease, allergies, etc.

3. Consumer Information

There are now several programs and campaigns launched by the government and various health sectors to provide information to people on how to apply wellness solutions. You will find programs that encourage people to drive sober, stay away from recreational drugs and harmful substances or stay safe in the workplace. There are also programs and groups that help people successfully get off vices like smoking, drug abuse and alcoholism. People will be able to know the symptoms and consequences of each, as well as the related diseases that can progress if they do not change their lifestyle.

4. Business Opportunities

This is also a perfect time to start businesses that focus on preventive health care. These financial opportunities prove to be more effective and sustainable compared to running establishments that only offer palliative and symptomatic care. Examples are MLMs or multilevel marketing companies that offer all-natural supplements, drinks and boosters that detoxify and enhance the immune system.

There are also establishments that help people stay on the lifestyle program, such as spas, gyms and stress management centers. People usually invest in programs that cleanse their bodies and get rid of stress such as getting a massage, doing yoga and breathing exercises or hiring a nutritionist. Individuals themselves can set up their own business to spread the advantages of wellness solutions and fight disease.

Wellness Solutions for Disease Prevention

Most doctors and experts will agree that taking the precautionary measures that will prevent disease and avoid further complications to existing ones is key to having a long and healthy life. People should be more aware and informed of the advantages that come with diagnostic procedures and taking the right steps that will keep them free of illness, regardless of their medical and family history. Even those who are already suffering from certain conditions can get treated quickly and avoid further problems.

Classifying the Preventive Methods

Three experts of disease prevention and use of substances, namely Gorden, Baxley and Kumpfer, presented a three-level classification system for prevention methods. The three levels are defined as universal, selective and indicated prevention. These classes have been accepted and are used by various groups and institutions such as the NIDA, the United States Institute of Medicine and the European Monitoring Centre for Drugs and Drug Addiction.

Aside from the three-tier model, another approach called environmental prevention is also applied. The approach focuses on the community and is based on methods that prevent drug and substance abuse. Some of the approaches used in environmental prevention include bans and prohibition of unhealthy habits like alcohol advertising, smoking in designated areas and drug campaigns. Actions at the micro and macro level are also used widely, such as drug tests, student drug testing, roadside sobriety and providing fines and warnings for related offenses.

Describing the Levels

Universal Prevention covers entire populations, such as schools, cities, countries, communities, etc. and focuses on the delay or prevention of drug, alcohol and tobacco abuse. All individuals are given the proper skills and information required to avoid the problem, without any screening or tests. The second level, selective prevention, covers groups of individuals with the risk of growing problems due to alcohol dependence or abuse. These individuals are more likely to develop diseases and health problems and the habit can stem and be distinguished by factors like family history, gender, age and financial well-being. An example is setting drug campaigns that add information and awareness.

The third level is indicated prevention, which includes a screening process and plans to identify people that show early signs of drug or alcohol abuse, aside from other odd behaviors. Some of the things that indicate the problem include failing marks among students, disorderly conduct, alienation from family and friends and identified problem consumption.

Targeting Everyone

People do not need to be described as a substance abuser or at high risk for developing unhealthy habits and serious disease before preventive methods can be done. In fact, government and health sectors try to implement and intervene in groups that are categorized as healthy and relatively disease-free. This promotes the idea of wellness solutions so that people can be aware of the consequences and can fully identify themselves in the class if they notice any change or symptom. The approaches can target whole communities or individuals depending on the classified level. Regardless of the scope and extent of the preventive practice, the goal is to reduce the risks and promote well-being.